COLLATERAL DAMAGE:

The Mental Health Effects of the Pandemic

Carla Mooney

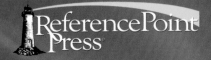

San Diego, CA

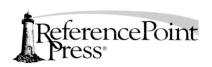

About the Author

Carla Mooney is the author of many books for young adults and children. She lives in Pittsburgh, Pennsylvania, with her husband and three children.

For more information, contact:
ReferencePoint Press, Inc.
PO Box 27779
San Diego, CA 92198
www.ReferencePointPress.com

Picture Credits:

Cover: Xesai/iStock
6: Shutterstock.com
10: Suzanne Tucker/Shutterstock.com
12: Prostock-studio/Shutterstock.com
15: iStock
19: Micha Weber/Shutterstock.com
22: Ringo Chiu/Shutterstock.com
25: coldsnowstorm/iStock

28: kjophoto/iStock
32: insta_photos/Shutterstock.com
38: Human Age/iStock
41: insta_photos/Shutterstock.com
45: Filip Jedraszak/Shutterstock.com
49: Human Role/iStock
51: lev radin/Shutterstock.com
53: Quisquilia/Shutterstock.com

LIBRARY OF CONGRESS CATALOGING-IN-PUBLICATION DATA

Names: Mooney, Carla, 1970- author.
Title: Collateral damage : the mental health effects of the pandemic / by Carla Mooney.
Description: San Diego, CA : ReferencePoint Press, 2022. | Includes bibliographical references and index.
Identifiers: LCCN 2020056766 (print) | LCCN 2020056767 (ebook) | ISBN 9781678200763 (library binding) | ISBN 9781678200770 (ebook)
Subjects: LCSH: COVID-19 (Disease)--United States. | COVID-19 (Disease)--Psychological aspects--United States--Juvenile literature. | COVID-19 (Disease)--Economic aspects--United States--Juvenile literature.
Classification: LCC RA644.C672 M66 2022 (print) | LCC RA644.C672 (ebook) | DDC 362.1962/414--dc23
LC record available at https://lccn.loc.gov/2020056766
LC ebook record available at https://lccn.loc.gov/2020056767

Missing Life

When the coronavirus pandemic hit the United States in early 2020, many people hunkered down in their homes to slow the virus's spread. At first, A.P. (who uses her initials for privacy) embraced the opportunity to work from her Washington, DC, home and slow down from her typical busy schedule as a lawyer. Like many people, A.P. used some of her newfound downtime for cooking, crafts, and gardening while she stayed alone in her apartment. Initially, she enjoyed the relaxed days and having time for her hobbies.

Yet as the weeks of isolation dragged on, A.P. found herself missing her busy life. She missed meeting coworkers and friends at restaurants and bars. Isolated and lonely, A.P. struggled with depression, a condition that she had experienced in the past. "My energy levels were really low," she says. "There were full days where I couldn't get myself to do any sort of work."[1] Being isolated also made it easier for A.P. to ignore warning signs about her mental health. "I didn't have anybody else who was working in the space, so it was like I had no one else to see me not work. I was able to pretend that things were fine for way longer than I think my friends who live with others were able to,"[2] she says.

The virus that forced A.P. and millions of others to stay home for months on end is a new type of coronavirus. It spreads primarily through saliva droplets or nasal discharge when an infected person speaks, sneezes, sings, or coughs. Many who contract the virus experience mild to moderate symptoms, including cough, fever, shortness of breath, body aches, sore throat, loss of taste or smell, gastrointestinal distress, headache, and congestion. Hundreds of thousands of others have become severely ill with COVID-19, the disease caused by the virus. By the end of 2020, according to the Johns Hopkins Coronavirus Resource Center, more than 345,000 people in the United States had died of COVID-19. The number of deaths worldwide exceeded 1.8 million. Both numbers continued to rise into 2021.

In an attempt to slow the spread of the highly contagious virus, countries worldwide implemented a variety of public health measures. At first, many countries closed their borders, schools, and businesses. They instituted lockdowns and ordered citizens to stay at home—for weeks or months at a time. When communities began to reopen, many governments required citizens to wear masks and practice social distancing, restricted the operation of schools and some businesses, and limited the size of public and private gatherings.

Mental Health Fallout

Throughout 2020 and into the early months of 2021, coronavirus infection rates and COVID-19 hospitalizations and deaths rose, fell, and rose again. In many places, businesses that had opened, even if only for limited service, were again forced to close. Many schools that had started bringing students back into the classroom went back to online learning. Daily life did not return to normal.

All the while mental health experts were warning of another looming crisis—the mental health fallout from the pandemic. According to an October 2020 report from Mental Health America (MHA), the number of people seeking mental health help increased by 93 percent for anxiety and 62 percent for depression from 2019 to 2020. In addition to more people seeking help, the level of distress was also more pronounced. The report noted a troubling increase in thoughts of suicide and self-harm.

For teens and young adults, the mental health strain of the pandemic has also been significant. According to the MHA report, the rate of youth ages eleven to seventeen who reported needing mental health support rose 9 percent over pre-pandemic 2019 levels. This age group was also more likely than any other age group to experience more severe depression and anxiety.

MHA president Paul Gionfriddo notes that his organization has seen heightened levels of anxiety and depression among all age groups since the pandemic began. He says:

> This is a troubling trend being fueled by loneliness and isolation. We are also seeing alarming numbers of children [ages eleven to seventeen] reporting thoughts of suicide and self-harm. We already knew that not enough was being done to support people living with mental illness, but the State of Mental Health in America report confirms the trend that mental health in the U.S. continues to get worse.[3]

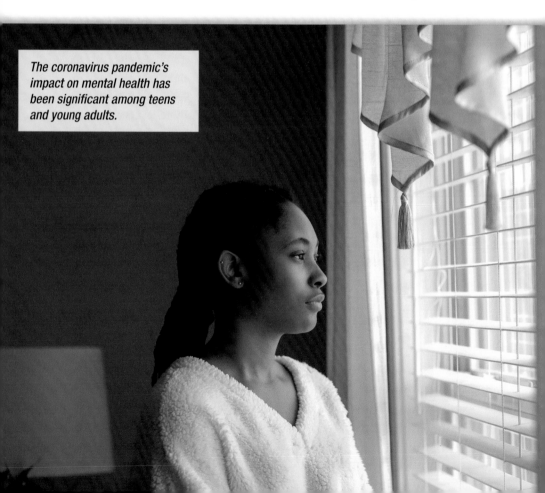

The coronavirus pandemic's impact on mental health has been significant among teens and young adults.

Declining mental health during the pandemic has not been a problem only in the United States. In countries worldwide, people have struggled with isolation, loss of income, grief, and fear. Recognizing this problem, the United Nations warned countries to take the pandemic's impact on mental health seriously. "COVID-19 has interrupted essential mental health services around the world just when they're needed most," says Tedros Adhanom Ghebreyesus, World Health Organization director-general. He urged world leaders to not neglect the mental health needs of their populations, adding, "Good mental health is absolutely fundamental to overall health and well-being."[4]

> "COVID-19 has interrupted essential mental health services around the world just when they're needed most."[4]
>
> —Tedros Adhanom Ghebreyesus, World Health Organization director-general

Isolated and Lonely

When the pandemic surged in the United States in early 2020, Lindsey Hornickel, a twenty-five-year-old living in Louisville, Kentucky, believed she could manage. Although she had struggled with depression in the past, Hornickel's mental health seemed to be good. With some of the extra time she had on her hands, she took on more work from home. She reassured herself that everything would be fine and refused to dwell on any potential worries.

Months into the pandemic and its social isolation, Hornickel's mental health suddenly plummeted. "I went through a depressive swing. It was unbearable,"[5] she says. Eventually, it got so bad that Hornickel confessed to her roommate she was having suicidal thoughts. She entered a treatment program to deal with her depression, bipolar disorder, and suicidal thoughts. Although Hornickel improved with treatment, she worried about sliding back into depression and suicidal thoughts as the pandemic continued to drag on. "For me, personally, the nighttime is really hard," Hornickel says. "And when there's not sunlight and sunshine and things to do—at that time in the winter—it definitely compounds those feelings."[6]

Hornickel was not alone in feeling isolated, lonely, and depressed. Research shows that difficulties with mental health have been increasing since the beginning of the pandemic. Mental health experts believe that measures taken to protect public health and reduce the spread of the coronavirus, such as lockdowns and social distancing, have had a devastating impact on mental health.

Mental Health Struggles on the Rise

Lockdowns, masks, and social distancing were aimed at slowing the virus's spread. When people adhered to these measures, infections slowed, but feelings of isolation and loneliness grew. People found their regular social routines disrupted. In many cases they no longer went to school or work. They could not meet friends for dinner at restaurants or work out at their gyms. Youth, high school, and college sports canceled entire seasons. Without their normal social routines, people could only interact with a small, limited group of people. While many people attempted to connect with family and friends virtually, the physical separation and isolation made it more difficult to make meaningful social connections. As a result, many people felt increasingly lonely and isolated. "We are social creatures—designed to eye gaze, handhold, laugh—and our bodies and brains are rewarded when we do this," says Dara Schwartz, a clinical psychologist. "When we don't or feel we can't, we do not feel like ourselves."[7]

Before the pandemic began, British artist Capella regularly spent hours alone during the week to paint and work on her art. On the weekends, Capella socialized, mingling and talking with friends and strangers in local restaurants and stores. The pandemic ended that routine. Capella found herself isolated without her usual social routine. "It's been really difficult . . . because such a big part of my life was just talking to strangers and meeting new people, but now it feels like that has all been put on hold," she says. "I've been alone before, but this loneliness is new."[8]

"It's been really difficult . . . because such a big part of my life was just talking to strangers and meeting new people, but now it feels like that has all been put on hold. I've been alone before, but this loneliness is new."[8]

—Capella, a British artist

Loneliness Affects Mental Health

Social isolation and loneliness affect everyone in different ways. Some people can adjust to these changes, while others have a hard time doing that. For the latter group, loneliness can increase anxiety and depression. For Mary Kathryn Kimray of Raleigh, North Carolina, the isolation and social distancing required during the pandemic left her feeling stressed and overwhelmed. As her anxiety worsened, Kimray talked to her doctor, who suggested she seek help from a therapist. Through several virtual appointments, Kimray learned how to calm her anxiety.

Research shows that the isolation and loneliness of the pandemic have had a significant effect on mental health. When Boston University researchers compared the results of a study done in 2017–2018 with their own new study, conducted in 2020, they found a threefold increase in depression among American adults.

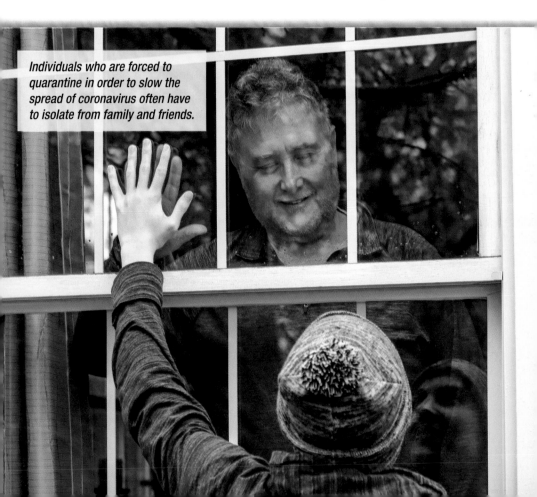

Individuals who are forced to quarantine in order to slow the spread of coronavirus often have to isolate from family and friends.

Fighting Loneliness in Older Adults

The risk of experiencing severe illness from COVID-19 increases with age. As a result, older adults have been advised to socially isolate as much as possible during the pandemic. As months of little social interaction stretched through 2020 into 2021, social distancing and self-quarantining limited older adults' exposure to infection but did so at the cost of increased feelings of isolation and loneliness. Even before the pandemic, research showed that an estimated 25 percent of adults over age sixty-five were socially isolated. Under pandemic restrictions, that number has likely increased a great deal, causing concern among health experts. Aside from increases in anxiety, depression, and suicide, loneliness and isolation can lead to heightened risk of dementia, heart disease, stroke, and premature death.

The researchers said they expected to find an increase in depression, but they were surprised by how much it had changed. "We knew that poor mental health increased after large-scale events, based on previous research," says the study's lead researcher, Catherine Ettman of Boston University. "We were surprised at the high levels of depression; these rates were higher than what we have seen in the general population after other large-scale traumas like September 11th, Hurricane Katrina, and the Hong Kong unrest."[9]

Not only is depression more widespread, it has also become more intense for many people. The Boston University study found higher levels of depression symptoms across all demographic groups. "There were fewer people who had no depressive symptoms, and there were more people who had mild, moderate, moderately severe and severe depression symptoms,"[10] says Ettman.

Mental health professionals are seeing an increase in patients seeking help with depression and other mental health problems. The Disaster Distress Helpline, which offers counseling and emotional support, reported a staggering 335 percent increase in calls from March through July 2020 compared to the same period in 2019. "Helpline counselors have reported callers expressing feelings of isolation and interpersonal concerns related to physical

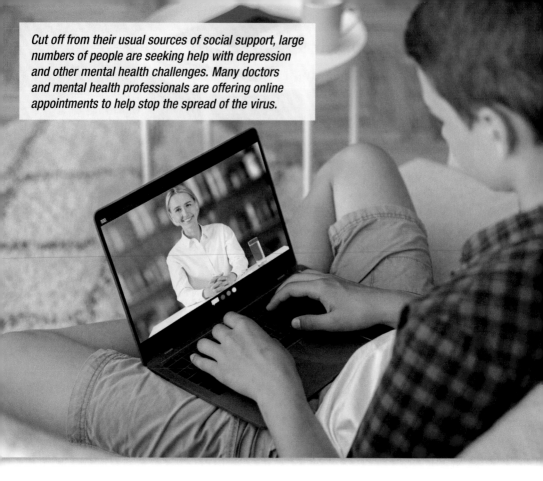

distancing such as being cut off from social supports,"[11] says Hannah Collins, a spokeswoman for Vibrant Emotional Health, which runs the helpline.

In Chicago, Cityscape Counseling has hired two new therapists since the pandemic began to handle the increased demand for counseling services. "We see a lot of single young professionals. I think it's been especially tough on them. The isolation, lack of connection, often enhances depression,"[12] says executive director Chelsea Hudson.

Before the pandemic, twenty-seven-year-old Olivia worked a flexible job that allowed her to travel the world. After the pandemic arrived, Olivia found herself stuck in her New York City apartment alone with little to do. Feeling trapped and lonely, she began to experience depression symptoms. "I just started to cry over everything. I was extra sensitive to the dumbest things—very,

very small things that normally, I don't think I'd have the time to be bothered by,"[13] she says. Olivia became lethargic and slept much more than usual. When she was not sleeping or crying, she often felt miserable and angry. When Olivia described her symptoms to a social worker, she was told that she was probably experiencing depression.

Panic and Anxiety

For some, feelings of stress, isolation, and loneliness have triggered bouts of anxiety. Melissa Cella, a wife and mother of two, had received therapy for panic attacks in the past. The pandemic's day-to-day isolation from extended family and friends led to increased anxiety and a return of her panic attacks. "If you go through a full blown anxiety attack, the next day you feel like you got the coronavirus—your throat hurts from hyperventilating and doing a weird breathing situation," she says. "It's different for everybody. I had a sore throat and my body was aching and my chest was tight."[14]

As the pandemic wore on, more people were reporting anxiety and panic attacks similar to what Cella was experiencing. "We have seen both an increase in people calling in for panic attacks and even calling for other things like anxiety . . . related to quarantine, social distancing, not having control of their lives,"[15] says Amanda Patterson, a mental health specialist.

Difficult-to-Manage Mental Illness

People who struggled with mental illness before the pandemic have been doubly challenged during this period. Naomi, a twenty-one-year-old psychology student, struggled with anxiety before the pandemic but was usually able to manage her condition by doing volunteer work and regularly getting out of the house. These coping techniques have not been available to her during the pandemic, leaving her feeling socially isolated and anxious. She has turned to journal writing in an effort to calm her thoughts.

Although the coronavirus pandemic has affected people in countries worldwide, a recent survey shows that Americans feel the mental health effects more than citizens of other countries. In a study published in August 2020, the Commonwealth Fund and survey research firm SSRS interviewed more than eight thousand adults age eighteen and older from the United States and nine other high-income countries. In the survey, one-third of US adults reported feeling stress, anxiety, and great sadness that they found challenging to manage alone. In comparison, less than one-quarter of adults from other countries reported similar feelings

To explain this difference, some mental health experts point to what they call "an epidemic of loneliness." Even before the COVID-19 pandemic, changes in American family life, work life, and social interaction were leading to rising social isolation and loneliness. The pandemic has intensified these feelings, as many people were only able to socialize with members of their own household for months at a time. For the millions of Americans who live alone, that led to months with few opportunities for meaningful social contact.

A November 2020 survey of people like Naomi who were already living with depression and anxiety confirmed that the constraints of life during the pandemic have added to the difficulty of coping with these conditions. Sixty-two percent of survey participants said that lack of motivation, panic attacks, self-harm thoughts, and other symptoms had worsened. In the survey, which was conducted by the GoodRx research team, participants identified stay-at-home orders and the resulting isolation and loneliness they experienced as strong factors for their growing depression and anxiety. In fact, more than 70 percent of those who said they quarantined for more than one week reported their depression and anxiety symptoms were worse, as compared to 53 percent who quarantined for less than a week. Tori Marsh, one of the study's authors and director of research at GoodRx, warns that the pandemic may have a long-lasting impact on mental health "well beyond the pandemic." She adds, "It's going to take a while for us to get fully back on our feet."[16]

Fending Off Isolation

To fend off the effects of social distancing, quarantine, and isolation, people across the country have developed creative ways to connect with others. Videoconferencing platforms like Zoom, FaceTime, and Google Hangouts have exploded in popularity. People use video technology to hold work meetings, attend online classes, and connect with family and friends. "With the technologies we have available today, we can stay home and protect against COVID-19, but still remain socially connected with people we love and care about via text, phone call, video and many other platforms,"[17] says Leah Welch, a psychologist at Scripps Health.

College student Allie Ouendag began doing video chats each week with friends to keep connected when they are unable to get together in person. "My scheduled weekly Zoom call with my friends has become a source of comfort and something I can look

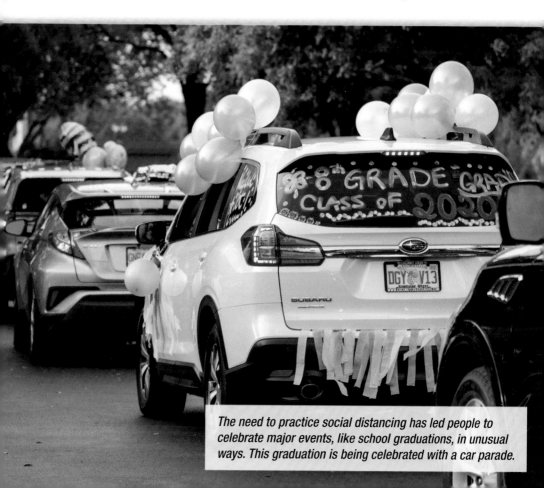

The need to practice social distancing has led people to celebrate major events, like school graduations, in unusual ways. This graduation is being celebrated with a car parade.

forward to during a hard week," she says. When one of her friends had a birthday, the group celebrated online with a virtual birthday cake and presents delivered by Amazon. "Zoom has bridged the distance beyond stay-at-home orders to allow for much need-ed social interactions and support to occur. Specifically in stressful situations, supporting one another is key to maintaining a healthy mindset,"[18] says Ouendag.

Some people have reimagined favorite activities to take advantage of outdoor space, where people could socially connect and still follow social distancing guidelines. Some people celebrated birthdays and graduations with parades of decorated cars with honking horns and flashing lights. Others held socially distant picnics, drive-in movies, and other outside activities where small groups of people could spread out and be safe. "We are, by nature, social primates, so it makes sense that being with other people helps us feel happier," says Laurie Santos, a psychology professor at Yale University. Sharing activities and seeking out ways to connect can provide an essential boost to mental health. "People are engaging in lots of intentional activities like Zoom dinners and socially distanced hikes with friends," says Santos. "If we're creative, social isolation doesn't have to mean social disconnection."[19]

> "Zoom has bridged the distance beyond stay-at-home orders to allow for much needed social interactions and support to occur. Specifically in stressful situations, supporting one another is key to maintaining a healthy mindset."[18]
>
> —Allie Ouendag, a college student

CHAPTER TWO

Money Worries

When the COVID-19 pandemic swept through the United States, Chan Tran was working in New York City and living with her husband in a tiny 700-square-foot (65 sq. m) apartment. The initial public health measures such as stay-at-home orders and lockdowns implemented to contain the spread of COVID-19 shuttered many businesses and devastated entire industries. Without a steady income stream, many employers were forced to lay off or furlough employees. When Tran's employer notified her that she was being furloughed from her corporate job, she was not surprised. Even so, the news hit her hard. The fear and anxiety she already felt about contracting the virus—and becoming severely ill or dying from it—was now magnified by fear and anxiety over being unemployed. "For a week, I'd randomly burst into tears. I sobbed while talking to my husband, cooking dinner, texting my friends, in the shower, and even when trying to go for a run to clear my head,"[20] she says.

Tran and her husband were not prepared to lose her income. She worried about how they would afford their rent, credit card payments, and large student loan payments that were due. She felt anxious and depressed. "I was having an existential breakdown," she says. "Rational me knew that losing my job was not a reflection of my performance or talent or skill set. Yet, I couldn't shake the feelings of worthlessness. That I had somehow failed. Unemployment is one of the scariest prospects in life. Losing your job can make you feel like you've lost your identity, which in turn could lead to a loss of self-worth."[21]

Economic Disaster

While public health measures such as lockdowns and social distancing were implemented to slow the coronavirus spread, these measures have also caused extreme financial difficulties for millions of people. Shutdowns and restrictions on businesses caused sales to plummet. In many cases, to stay afloat, companies were forced to lay off or furlough employees or cut their hours. Even after the initial shutdowns ended, demand for services in many industries was slow to return. Many people remained cautious about resuming their everyday social routines of eating out in restaurants, going to concerts, traveling, and more. As infections, hospitalizations, and deaths rose through 2020 and into 2021, businesses struggled to operate under changing restrictions, and many communities endured repeated cycles of closing and opening.

For many businesses, the pandemic's economic effects have been disastrous. High-interaction businesses such as restaurants, hotels, theaters, casinos, conference and event centers, and cruise lines struggled to reopen fully. Some were unable to recover and have closed their doors permanently. In Henderson County, North Carolina, Flat Rock Pizza announced in October 2020 that it would be closing. After twenty-two years in business, the owners made the difficult decision to shut down operations for good. "After losing money for several months, you have to stop the bleeding," says owner Jeannie Honeycutt. According to Honeycutt, the pandemic's economic burden was too great to overcome. "My heart is actually broken," she says.[22]

Losing Jobs and Income

As businesses and industries faced severe financial losses, millions of people across the United States lost their jobs and income sources. According to the Congressional Research Service, in the United States unemployment peaked in April 2020 at 14.7 percent, a level not seen in generations. Although that situation improved as the year progressed, many people were still without work. By September half of adults who reported losing their jobs

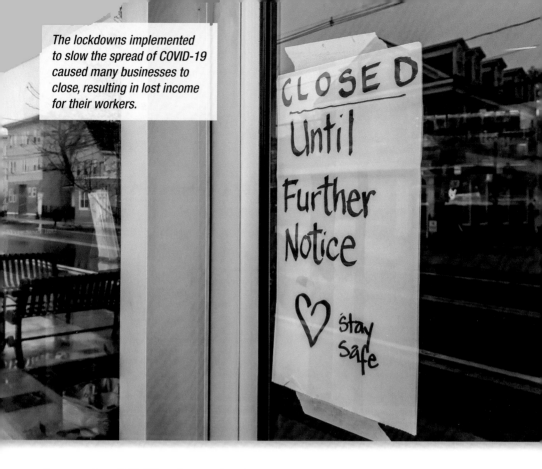

The lockdowns implemented to slow the spread of COVID-19 caused many businesses to close, resulting in lost income for their workers.

due to the COVID-19 pandemic were still unemployed, according to a Pew Research Center study. Among those who still had their jobs, the study notes, 60 percent said they were making less money because of wage cuts, reduced hours, or reduced demand for their work.

For many individuals and families, job losses and reduced wages bring extreme financial hardship. People in this position have struggled to pay their rent or mortgage—and some have been threatened with eviction. They have put off paying credit card bills and making payments on car loans and school loans. In some cases they have postponed medical treatment or delayed refilling prescriptions. Many have struggled to come up with enough money to pay for food. Under these conditions, stress, anxiety, and depression have grown. "We're seeing skyrocketing rates of job losses and food insecurity and stress," says Anna Johnson, a developmental psychologist at Georgetown University. "I think it will be very hard for these families who've lost income and jobs to get back to where they were. I think there will just be a lot of stress and turmoil in the household for the foreseeable future . . . that takes a toll."[23]

Financial Stress and Mental Health

Even before the coronavirus pandemic, financial concerns were among the leading causes of stress for Americans. For many people the pandemic's widespread job and income losses have intensified the financial pressures they face, putting them at greater risk for mental health problems. Research shows that job loss is linked to increased depression, anxiety, and low self-esteem. According to a July 2020 poll conducted by the Kaiser Family Foundation, households that experienced job or income loss reported higher adverse mental health due to worry and stress (58 percent) than households that did not have job or income loss (50 percent).

> "I think it will be very hard for these families who've lost income and jobs to get back to where they were. I think there will just be a lot of stress and turmoil in the household for the foreseeable future . . . that takes a toll."[23]
>
> —Anna Johnson, a developmental psychologist at Georgetown University

Khristan Yates understands these feelings. Before the pandemic, she worked as a quality assurance analyst at a marketing company—and she loved her job. Because she was earning a decent amount of money, she felt comfortable moving into a more spacious Chicago apartment with her two children. Then the pandemic swept through the United States. Like many businesses, Yates's employer struggled financially, and Yates was laid off. Losing her job made Yates feel like someone had pulled the floor out from underneath her. Without her income, she struggled to pay bills and buy enough food for her family. "I went from having a very stable stream of income and being OK to being very not OK," she says. The financial stress has caused Yates's anxiety to skyrocket. On

The Pandemic's Disproportionate Economic Impact

Many people have lost jobs or income because of the coronavirus pandemic. However, job and income losses have not been experienced equally across all demographic groups. According to the Brookings Institution, Hispanic, low-income, and young adults (ages eighteen to twenty-four) have experienced the highest rates of job and income loss compared to other demographic groups. The pandemic's job and income losses have likely hit these groups harder because they are more likely to work in industries devastated by the coronavirus, such as construction and hospitality.

In addition, some demographic groups have experienced a greater proportion of financial hardships related to the coronavirus pandemic, according to the Brookings Institution. As expected, low-income households were more likely to experience financial hardship than moderate-, middle-, and high-income households. However, race and ethnicity are also factors. Compared to White households, Black households have been more likely to have trouble paying rent, mortgage, and other bills. Hispanic households have been more likely to experience food insecurity than White households.

many days she struggles to get out of bed and sometimes forgets to eat. "I would make food for my children, of course, but when it came down to like me sitting down and eating, it didn't even register," she says. "So I would get up with headaches before the morning and [realize] 'oh well, you haven't eaten in two or three days. That's why your head is on fire.'"[24]

Amy Rivera, a single mother from Rochester, New York, also knows firsthand the anxiety that builds when a person loses his or her job. Before the pandemic, Rivera worked as a paraprofessional with special education students in the Rochester City School District. When schools across the country closed to limit the spread of the virus, Rivera's job ended. Without an income, she struggled to cover her expenses, including car payments, rent, and grocery bills. Rivera struggled to cope with the stress of this situation, and her worries escalated to the point that she was diagnosed with anxiety and depression. "I get anxiety and panic attacks every other day, and I don't take medication because the medication they give me tries to relax me, but it also

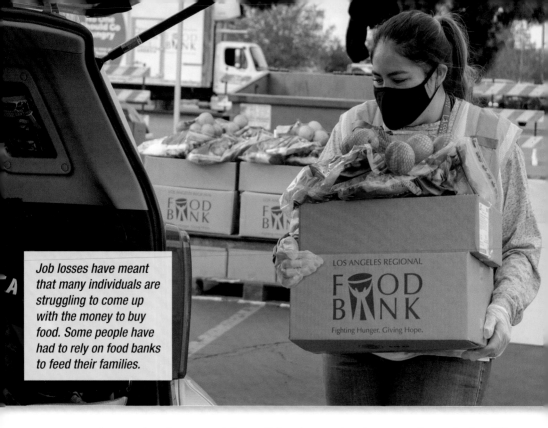

Job losses have meant that many individuals are struggling to come up with the money to buy food. Some people have had to rely on food banks to feed their families.

puts me to sleep and I can't be in my bed every day, all day,"[25] she says. Rivera hopes that when schools eventually resume in-person classes, she will be rehired for her old job. She is also looking into other job possibilities. Still, she admits that some days she feels overwhelmed and unable to cope with the financial stress. Yet she pushes through it for her sons. "I can't give up," she says. "because these kids, they need me."[26]

Losing a job not only means dealing with the financial impact of lost income and benefits. It can also mean the loss of one's identity. For many people, a job or career becomes an integral part of how they see themselves. "Work provides us time structure, it provides us identity, it provides us purpose, and it also provides us social interactions with others," says Connie Wanberg, an industrial and organizational psychologist at the University of Minnesota. "When you lose all that, it creates a lot of difficulties for people."[27]

Losing a job often triggers feelings of sadness and stress. Many people recover from these feelings and move on with their lives.

In some cases, these feelings can linger and develop into depression or anxiety. People having trouble dealing with job loss may find themselves preoccupied with thinking about the lost job. They may find it difficult to accept the loss or have feelings of bitterness toward their former employer. Some people may even struggle with feelings of worthlessness and the sense that life no longer has meaning without their former job.

> "Work provides us time structure, it provides us identity, it provides us purpose, and it also provides us social interactions with others. When you lose all that, it creates a lot of difficulties for people."[27]
>
> —Connie Wanberg, an industrial and organizational psychologist at the University of Minnesota

Worrying About the Future

Some of those still employed have also struggled emotionally and are worried about the future. They worry about losing their jobs or having their hours cut, as has happened to so many others. The constant uncertainty of the pandemic has increased stress and fear and led many people to experience serious bouts of anxiety even when their lives have seemed to be relatively stable.

Research by the University of Connecticut has confirmed this dynamic. "We definitely are seeing, within our employed participants, higher rates of anxiety than in individuals who indicated they were not employed,"[28] says researcher Natalie J. Shook. In their study published in September 2020, the researchers asked participants specific questions about their jobs and finances. The responses revealed that the pandemic has caused employed individuals to question the stability of their jobs and their financial status. The participants found it hard to plan for an uncertain future and predict what would happen to their jobs and finances over the next year, which caused an increase in anxiety and depression.

Increased Substance Use

Anxiety and depression resulting from job or income loss often lead to substance abuse. Many substances have been used to deaden emotional pain. "Alcohol is a very effective pain killer. But when it wears off, that pain comes back with a vengeance,"[29] says National Institute on Alcohol Abuse and Alcoholism director George Koob. Numerous research studies have shown a link between unemployment and substance use. Additionally, even the fear of losing a job can lead to increased use of alcohol, tobacco, and other substances. In some cases increased substance use can lead to addiction.

During the coronavirus pandemic, American adults have significantly increased their alcohol use, according to a study published in September 2020 by the Rand Corporation. The data show that Americans drank alcohol more frequently and in greater amounts in 2020 than in 2019. The study participants also reported that they had experienced more negative impacts, such as taking unnecessary risks or hurting their family due to their drinking.

Due to the study's findings, experts are concerned about how people deal with the stress, anxiety, and depression brought on by the pandemic. "The magnitude of these increases is striking," says Michael Pollard, the study's lead author and a sociologist at Rand. "People's depression increases, anxiety increases, [and] alcohol use

Game Over

In Asheville, North Carolina, the Well Played Board Game Café closed in October 2020 due to financial pressure caused by the coronavirus pandemic. "Things were going well, and then they took, of course, an immediate downturn," says Kevan Frazier, co-owner of the café. Before the pandemic, the café's customers would come in groups of four or more, pick a board game from the café's collection, and play for a couple of hours while eating and drinking. The groups sat close together and touched the same game pieces over and over. According to Frazier, the café's model no longer worked with the pandemic's social distancing rules. Even though the café did receive some federal and local grant money meant to help small businesses during the pandemic, it was not enough to pay its mounting debt. "The only way we could pay the bills would be to build more debt, and we would just reach a point that we had more debt than we would reasonably be able to pay off," Frazier says.

Quoted in Ryan Coulter, "2 More Mountain Businesses Forced to Close Because of Pandemic," WLOS.com (Asheville, NC), October 28, 2020. https://wlos.com.

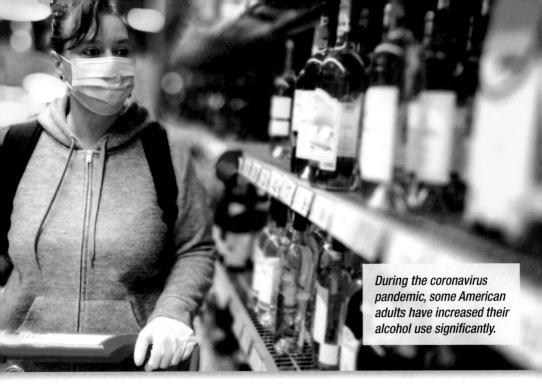

During the coronavirus pandemic, some American adults have increased their alcohol use significantly.

is often a way to cope with these feelings. But depression and anxiety are also the outcome of drinking; it's this feedback loop where it just exacerbates the problem that it's trying to address."[30]

As Joe Dinan's anxiety and stress built during the pandemic, he turned to alcohol as an escape. When Dinan lost his job in 2020, he felt hopeless and without a sense of purpose. These feelings led him to a familiar place: the liquor store and a bottle of vodka. Although he had been working for several years to control his drinking, the pandemic's stress drove him back to alcohol. "It got to a point when everything just compounded, and I didn't know what to do," he says. "We drink to hide from feelings, hide from life. We tend to isolate. Especially when addiction really gets advanced. Now people are isolated at home. And it presents a real challenge."[31]

For many people, the pandemic has caused extreme financial difficulties. As businesses have struggled through public health restrictions, workers have lost jobs and income. Businesses large and small have been forced to close. The crushing stress of financial worry can damage mental health, leading to increased anxiety, depression, and other mental health concerns.

CHAPTER THREE

The Mental Health Toll on Essential Workers

Ashli Hinds works two jobs: a package handler for a shipping company and a second job providing on-site tech support for an aerospace firm. During the pandemic, both positions were considered essential, and Hinds continued to go to work even when other businesses were closed. As an essential worker exposed to countless people daily, Hinds has been worried about her health and whether she will contract the coronavirus. Because she has diabetes (a preexisting condition), Hinds falls into a higher risk category of complications from the coronavirus. Hinds also worries about spreading the virus to friends and family. So when she does have time off work, she usually spends it alone. The constant strain and worry have impacted her mental health. "It is depression. It's like a monkey on my back," Hinds says. "Like I have nowhere to go, nobody to go see—and that's the hard part."[32]

Challenges for Essential Workers

During the pandemic, people who worked in jobs considered essential—such as health care workers, grocery store employees, delivery people, and factory workers—continued working. Avoiding contact with others was not an option, since their jobs could not be performed from home. These workers often faced shortages of personal protective equipment at work, such as masks, gowns, gloves, and more. Additionally, tests have been in short supply in many communities, and some essential workers were not able to get tested for the virus even if they were showing symptoms.

Like Hinds, many essential workers worried that they would be exposed to the coronavirus on the job due to unsafe working conditions. In fact, the number of COVID-19-related workplace safety complaints rose over 350 percent from mid-April to mid-August 2020, according to the Occupational Safety and Health Administration. Workers feared they would get sick and pass on the virus to family and friends, potentially causing serious illness. This stress and uncertainty have taken a serious toll on the mental health of essential workers. According to an August 2020 report from the Centers for Disease Control and Prevention (CDC), more than half of essential workers (54 percent) had experienced mental health issues during the pandemic—25 percent more than the general population.

While working as an intensive care nurse, Jess contracted COVID-19 during the spring of 2020. At first her symptoms were manageable, but she experienced intense shortness of breath and struggled to keep calm. "Suddenly I had visions of leaving my two children to grow up without me and I couldn't sleep through fear of not waking up. Climbing into an ambulance alone one night when it was particularly bad, genuinely feeling like there was a chance I wasn't coming home brought me stomach churning feelings I still can't shake from my mind," she says. Although Jess has physically recovered from COVID-19, she still struggles mentally. "I don't know how to explain it other than I constantly feel on edge. I'm so aware of my every breath that I'm most probably over breathing in my panic. I used to be able to sleep through the night with no problems . . . but I can't remember the last full night's sleep I had," she says. She is also having panic attacks. "The panic attacks are coming slightly less frequently, but every now and again my chest still goes tight, my heart starts beating like it's going to burst out of my chest and it

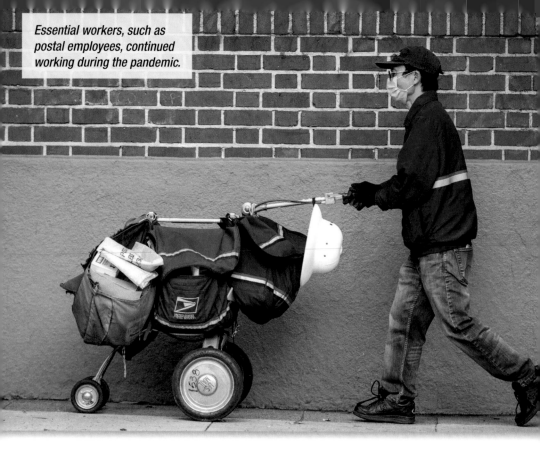

takes most of my strength to keep it together and just breathe through it until it passes. This crippling anxiety and the panic attacks that come with it are totally uncharted territory for me,"[33] she says.

Increasing Workloads and Burnout

In addition to fears of getting sick from the coronavirus, many essential workers have also been dealing with increasing pressures at work. Many have been required to take on extra responsibilities as coworkers call in sick due to illness or quit rather than expose themselves to infection on the job. Employers often could not or would not hire replacements, leaving remaining workers to shoulder the extra workload, often without additional pay and in risky working conditions.

Essential workers who deal with the public have also faced additional pressures that have not previously been part of the job. At grocery stores and big box retailers, essential workers have had to deal with confrontational customers. Anger over mask-wearing rules, limited availability of store stock, and long lines has sometimes turned ugly. Angry customers have taken out their frustrations on workers by yelling at them, insulting them, and in a few instances, shooting them.

> "This crippling anxiety and the panic attacks that come with it are totally uncharted territory for me."[33]
>
> —Jess, a nurse in an intensive care unit who contracted COVID-19

Terri Prunty Kay has worked for nearly a decade as a Walmart cashier near her home in Sonoma County, California. While she has had to deal with her share of angry customers in the past, it was never this bad. Now she has been forced to deal regularly with aggressive and angry customers. "It's been a nightmare," she says. "The first three months there were item limits. Everyone was angry and combative. Now it's the masks." She said the store was understaffed, which resulted in long lines at her register. "It's exhausting, mentally, emotionally and physically,"[34] she says.

As a result of the additional stress, workload, and responsibilities, burnout among essential workers has been rising. In August 2020, 58 percent of American workers reported feeling burned out, as compared to 45 percent in April 2020, according to a national poll conducted by Eagle Hill Consulting. In the poll, 35 percent of workers in August 2020 said that their burnout was related to COVID-19 circumstances, compared to 25 percent in April.

> "It's exhausting, mentally, emotionally and physically."[34]
>
> —Terry Prunty Kay, an essential worker

At Camp Lejeune, a US Marine Corps base in North Carolina, civilian workers in the base's food service halls have reported heightened pressures that have strained mental and emotional health. They described working short-staffed while being expected to keep up with full workloads. In September workers also told an interviewer that they feared getting sick because many marines on the base were ignoring social distancing guidelines and refused to wear masks. "The workload is so high that for the past three weeks alone we have lost seven employees who have just up and quit after working a day or two. Most of my coworkers have at one point in time broken down crying at work, myself included. It's gotten so bad that I usually cry before work, or in the bathroom after a particularly grueling shift,"[35] says one worker.

Additional Challenges for Health Care Workers

Health care workers have had to deal with their own share of challenges and stressors during the pandemic. They have faced repeated exposure to the virus as they treated patients, often while dealing with shortages of personal protective equipment. In addition to worrying about their own health, they have had to deal with increased workloads and responsibilities as coworkers call in sick due to illness or quarantine.

Also, many health care workers have been responsible for caring for extremely sick patients and dealing with a new virus for which treatments have been uncertain. Watching patients deteriorate despite trying every available medical treatment has made many health care workers feel helpless.

Adding to the stress, pandemic hospital rules have strictly limited and often banned visitors. Nurses and nursing assistants have been called upon to step in for families who cannot be at a dying patient's side. They hold the patient's hand, set up video calls between the patient and family members, and provide emotional support. "That's not normal," says Dr. Jessica Gold, an assistant professor of psychiatry at Washington University in St. Louis, Missouri. "And they're wearing this gear that creates a physical barrier, but you're then asking so much from them emotionally, to be there for everybody. So it's just a lot."[36]

At Christiana Hospital in Newark, Delaware, the stress of being the only person available to comfort a patient at the end of life was felt strongly by one young nurse as she sat with a seventy-five-year-old man dying from COVID-19. Because no family members were

For some essential workers, the strain of the coronavirus pandemic became too much to bear. Some came to believe that the only way to end their pain was suicide. According to an August 2020 report from the CDC, more than 20 percent of essential workers have thought about suicide. Some have acted on those feelings. During New York City's spring 2020 virus surge, Dr. Lorna Breen, an emergency room doctor with no history of mental illness, committed suicide. Before her death, Breen had spent weeks treating an overwhelming tide of coronavirus patients at her hospital. She contracted COVID-19 herself but returned to work in less than two weeks. Her father says that when he last talked to Breen, she seemed detached and not herself as she described a rush of coronavirus patients who were dying before hospital staff could even get them out of ambulances. "She tried to do her job, and it killed her," he says.

Quoted in Ali Watkins et al., "Top E.R. Doctor Who Treated Virus Patients Dies by Suicide," *New York Times*, April 27, 2020. www.nytimes.com.

allowed in his room, the nurse took their place during the man's final moments of life. Wearing full protective gear, she dimmed the room's lights and played quiet music. She held the man's hand and spoke softly to him. Then she held an iPad so he could see the face and hear the voice of a family member in the hospital hallway. After the man died, the nurse left the room and found a secluded spot to cry.

Increased Risk of Mental Health Issues

While health care workers have been praised for their work treating sick coronavirus patients, the job's strain has triggered mental health problems for many. Crushed under the stress of their jobs, health care workers have an increased risk of developing symptoms of depression, anxiety, post-traumatic stress disorder (PTSD), and other mental health conditions. If their mental health problems become severe enough, this could affect the health care workers' ability to be focused and effective on the job.

Studies of health care workers in countries worldwide have revealed the mental health impact of the coronavirus on these essential workers. In one study of Chinese health care workers published by the *Journal of the American Medical Association* in March 2020, investigators found that a significant number of health care workers who were directly involved in diagnosing, treating, or caring for COVID-19 patients had experienced symptoms of depression, anxiety, insomnia, and other distress. In May 2020 the World Health Organization issued a report on the pandemic's effects on mental health, emphasizing the enormous stresses placed on health care workers and the resulting vulnerabilities these workers have to mental health problems.

Jodie Gord works as a manager of patient care at Aurora St. Luke's Medical Center in Milwaukee, Wisconsin. As her hospital treated increasing numbers of COVID-19 patients, some of whom were on ventilators, Gord's feelings of helplessness have grown. As each new patient enters her intensive care unit, Gord worries

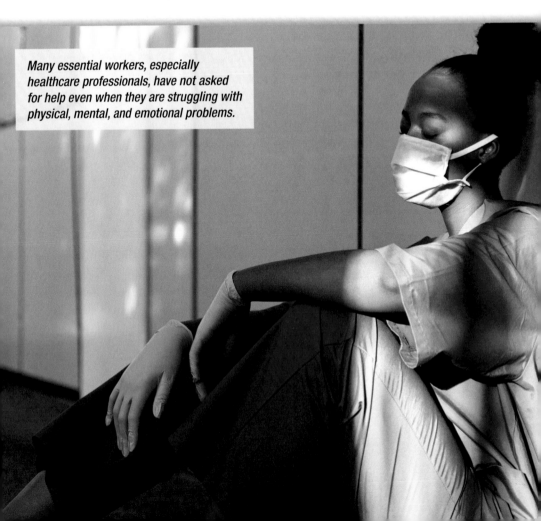

Many essential workers, especially healthcare professionals, have not asked for help even when they are struggling with physical, mental, and emotional problems.

that she will not be able to help them recover. The constant stress has taken a toll on her mental health. "Mentally, I was really going into a dark, slippery slope," Gord said in an October news interview. "In these last two weeks, I really felt it. And I felt it hard. I would be at home and just start crying for no reason."[37] To help herself and her co-workers deal with their feelings, Gord placed a journal in the staff room. In the journal, doctors and nurses who care for very sick COVID-19 patients write their thoughts and vent their feelings. In one entry, an overwhelmed health care worker wrote about feeling defeated by the seemingly endless struggle: "Anxiety and depression have been kicking my butt lately."[38]

> "Mentally, I was really going into a dark, slippery slope. In these last two weeks, I really felt it. And I felt it hard. I would be at home and just start crying for no reason."[37]
>
> —Jodi Gord, manager of patient care at Aurora St. Luke's Medical Center in Milwaukee, Wisconsin

Fear of Infecting Loved Ones

Many essential workers worry that they will become infected with COVID-19 while at work and in contact with other people. Not only are they concerned about their own health, but many are also terrified that they will bring the virus home and infect vulnerable family and friends. To protect their loved ones, some essential workers have decided to isolate themselves from family to prevent spreading the virus.

Dr. Andrew Cohen, an emergency medicine doctor in Paterson, New Jersey, fears that he might have brought COVID-19 home to his family. His in-laws lived with him, his wife, and their two children. In March 2020 both of his in-laws became seriously ill with the virus and were admitted to the hospital, where both died. The guilt Cohen feels over their deaths can sometimes be overwhelming. "Did I bring this virus into my house?"[39] he asks. In the hours before his next shift at work begins, Cohen becomes anxious and foggy. He wonders if he will become the next person in his household to die from the coronavirus. After each shift, he performs a meticulous cleaning ritual that even he describes as excessive. Only then will he allow himself to be near his family.

Cohen worries about his own mental health. How long will he feel compelled to perform this cleaning ritual? How long will it take for his fear of the coronavirus infecting him or his family to fade? And if and when he reaches out for help, will anyone be able to respond? "We've always been told to suck it up and move on. Will there be people there to help us?"[40] he asks.

Hard to Ask for Help

Many essential workers, particularly those who work in health care, have not asked for help even though they are struggling physically, mentally, and emotionally. "Physicians are often very self-reliant and may not easily ask for help. In this time of crisis,

PTSD in Health Care Workers

The enormous mental, emotional, and even physical stress the pandemic has placed on frontline health care workers may put them at risk of developing PTSD. PTSD is a mental health disorder triggered by experiencing or witnessing a terrifying event. A person with PTSD may experience uncontrolled thoughts about the event, severe anxiety, nightmares, and flashbacks. Sometimes, soldiers who experience or see horrific events on the battlefield struggle with PTSD after returning home.

Mental health experts like Shauna Springer, a psychologist who treats patients with trauma-related mental conditions, warn that health care workers treating COVID-19 patients face an increased risk of PTSD. Springer says:

Many of the war fighters I have worked with are physicians. They are now on the front lines of the COVID outbreak. They are telling me this trauma is worse than even many of the combat zones they have been in. . . . The healthcare workers on the front lines are the new warriors. The kind of trauma they are facing is very similar to what active duty service members and veterans have experienced for years.

Quoted in Relias Media, "Watch for PTSD in Healthcare Workers Following Their Covid-19 Experience," July 1, 2020. www.reliasmedia.com.

with high workload and many uncertainties, this trait can add to the load that they carry internally," says Dr. Chantal Brazeau, a psychiatrist at the Rutgers New Jersey Medical School. As the pandemic stretched on for months, mental health experts warned that medical and other essential workers have been left to deal with their emotions, which may worsen over time. "As the pandemic intensity seems to fade, so does the adrenaline. What's left are the emotions of dealing with the trauma and stress of the many patients we cared for," says Dr. Mark Rosenberg, chair of the emergency department at St. Joseph's Health in Paterson, New Jersey. "There is a wave of depression, letdown, true PTSD, and a feeling of not caring anymore that is coming."[41]

Throughout the pandemic, essential workers have provided the care, products, and services that people across the country desperately need. In doing so, they have put their own lives and those of their family and friends at risk. As the stress on these workers has grown, so has the threat to their mental health.

> "As the pandemic intensity seems to fade, so does the adrenaline. What's left are the emotions of dealing with the trauma and stress of the many patients we cared for. There is a wave of depression, letdown, true PTSD, and a feeling of not caring anymore that is coming."[41]
>
> —Dr. Mark Rosenberg, chair of the emergency department at St. Joseph's Health in Paterson, New Jersey

CHAPTER FOUR

Vulnerable Teens and Young Adults

Fourteen-year-old Aya Raji was a typical New York City teenager before the pandemic. She filled her days with school, after-school clubs and activities, and visits with friends. When the coronavirus spread through the city, Raji's Brooklyn school switched from in-person classes to remote learning. The once busy teenager was now stuck at home, staring at her laptop as part of daily virtual classes. Many nights she had trouble sleeping as anxiety took over her thoughts. "I felt like I was trapped in my own little house and everyone was far away," Raji says. "When you're with friends, you're completely distracted and you don't think about the bad stuff going on. During the beginning of quarantine, I was so alone. All the sad things I used to brush off, I realized I couldn't brush them off anymore."[42]

Many people have had trouble dealing with social isolation during the pandemic. Teens like Raji have keenly felt the loss of connecting with friends and taking part in the rituals of middle school and high school. Although many schools reopened in the fall with a blend of in-person and remote learning, the required social distancing and masking rules still have made it difficult for young people to connect. "A lot of adults assume teens have it easy," Raji says. "But it's hitting us the hardest."[43]

Lives Disrupted

Like everyone else, the lives of teens and young adults have been upended by the pandemic. All of the typical things teens do—such as going to school, spending time with friends, shopping at the mall, and more—have either been taken away or changed significantly. Instead of in-person school, many students attend class virtually via a computer. School social activities such as sports, dances, club meetings, and charity events have been postponed or canceled outright to limit the coronavirus's spread. Even when young people can see their friends, they have been told to do it in a socially distant way, staying at least 6 feet (1.8 m) away from another person and wearing a mask.

> "A lot of adults assume teens have it easy. But it's hitting us the hardest."[43]
>
> —Aya Raji, a fourteen-year-old struggling with isolation during the pandemic

For Aaliyah Kelley, a seventeen-year-old high school senior from Campbell, California, the social isolation and stress she has endured during the pandemic have been challenging. Missing out on senior year activities that were canceled because of the pandemic was a big blow. Not seeing friends has been hard. Working as a part-time cashier at a local drug store has been unsettling when she finds herself on the receiving end of angry comments from customers who are frustrated by stock shortages or purchase limits. She says she has not seen her friends in months and finds it difficult to talk to them via text messages about her stress. Although Kelley tries to hold in her stress, it shows up anyway. "I pull my hair when I'm stressed out. I did see myself pulling my hair more,"[44] she admits.

The Struggle of Online Learning

In addition to the loss of social connections, many teens have struggled with the switch to online learning. This change has affected students of all abilities. Some have had problems focusing for hours at a time on a computer screen. Some have had difficulty

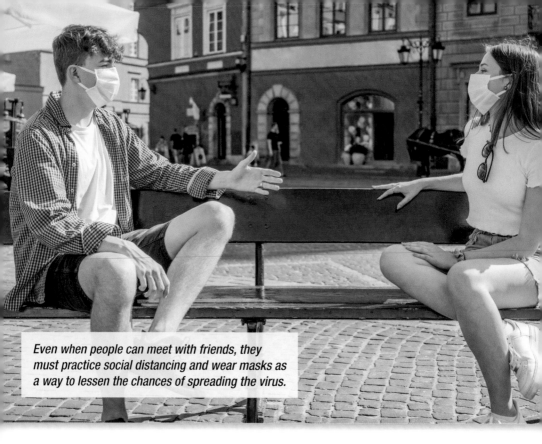

Even when people can meet with friends, they must practice social distancing and wear masks as a way to lessen the chances of spreading the virus.

asking questions remotely or have struggled to understand difficult topics without face-to-face help from teachers. Some students are less motivated to keep on top of assignments without the structure of in-person classes. Some students do not have access to computers, internet connections, or a quiet place to do schoolwork at home. In some cases students who used to do well academically have been falling behind. In other cases students who always struggled with academics are struggling even more. Many teens are unsure how or where to ask for help, adding to the stress and anxiety of life during the pandemic.

A series of student polls conducted by the University of North Texas (UNT) newspaper *North Texas Daily* in September 2020 revealed student worries about online learning. In the survey, 84 percent of UNT students admitted that they felt less motivated to complete assignments than when they attended in-person classes. The majority of students polled (64 percent) said it was more likely that they would fail a class in the fall 2020 semester.

For Ruby Rodriquez, a freshman at St. Anthony High School in Milwaukee, Wisconsin, online learning has made it significantly more difficult to learn and remain motivated. Instead of walking into a classroom while chatting with friends, Rodriquez now logs on to school via a laptop as she sits alone in her dining room. Most of the time, she cannot even see her classmates, since most of them keep their computer cameras turned off. Her teachers lecture for most the class period, and there is little student discussion or input. In this environment, Rodriquez has felt disconnected and isolated from her classmates and friends. She has missed turning in assignments, and her grades have suffered, dropping from As and Bs to Ds and Fs.

Worried About Family

Teens have also been struggling with the fear that loved ones will get sick and die or that their parents will lose their jobs, leaving the family with no money for food, rent, and other necessities. Not having their usual support systems of friends nearby has allowed these types of fears to grow.

Too Much Social Media

The upsides and downsides of social media have been laid bare during the pandemic. Social media has been a lifeline for many teens and young adults as they searched for ways to connect with others. But social media platforms have also bombarded users with a steady stream of dire headlines, disturbing news stories, and dangerous predictions.

Mental health experts have seen increases in anxiety and depression over the course of the pandemic—and they believe that social media has contributed to these feelings. To reduce this effect, experts have urged teens, young adults, and others to put down their phones and take regular breaks from social media. "We know that watching too much of this tends to make people pretty anxious. And focus on facts, not fear," says David Trotter, a licensed clinical psychologist. This time can be better put to use engaging with family, going outside, or doing other enjoyable activities.

Quoted in Texas Tech University Health Sciences Center, "How Social Media Affects Our Mental Health During a Pandemic," *Daily Dose* (blog), May 27, 2020. https://dailydose.ttuhsc.edu.

When eighteen-year-old Nicole DiMaio's mother fell sick with COVID-19, DiMaio became her mother's primary caregiver. Every day, she cleaned the house, took care of her younger sister, and cooked healthy food for the family. In between household responsibilities, DiMaio crammed in schoolwork. Every time her mother went to the emergency room for breathing treatments, DiMaio feared she might never return. In stressful situations, DiMaio would normally lean on her friends for comfort. Yet because of the pandemic, she could not see them in person. Instead, she connected with them on social media. But that was not enough. The stress and fear over her mother's health caused DiMaio's anxiety to surge. "Being 18 and taking it all in is a lot," she says. "My chest would get really heavy and everything inside my body would be jumping. The tears would start coming. I would hyperventilate and pace the house until my sister brought me back to reality and said, 'Hey you're here, relax.'"[45]

Hitting Mental Health Hard

Experts say the mental health impact of the pandemic has hit teens and young adults particularly hard. Several surveys of high school and college students reveal that their mental health has been negatively impacted by social isolation, money worries, and uncertainty surrounding their education and future careers. Young adults aged eighteen to twenty-four reported the highest level of anxiety and depression of any age group, according to an August 2020 CDC report on mental health during the pandemic. Nearly 63 percent of young adults reported symptoms of anxiety, depression, or both. Almost 75 percent of that group described at least one of their symptoms as significant.

In a separate study, researchers reported similar trends with students screening positive for anxiety and depression at higher rates than in previous years. This study was conducted by the Student Experience in the Research University (SERU) Consortium, a research collaboration among several universities and scholars. "It is clear that the COVID-19 pandemic has elevated the frequency with which students experience mental health disorders,"[46] says Krista Soria, assistant director for research and strategic partnerships for the SERU Consortium.

Sarah Suntheimer, a Kent State University student, knows firsthand how the pandemic has increased mental health problems in teens and young adults. Suntheimer, who was studying math and political science, has struggled with depression during the pandemic. During the 2020 spring semester, Suntheimer was

> "It is clear that the COVID-19 pandemic has elevated the frequency with which students experience mental health disorders."[46]
>
> —Krista Soria, assistant director for research and strategic partnerships for the SERU Consortium

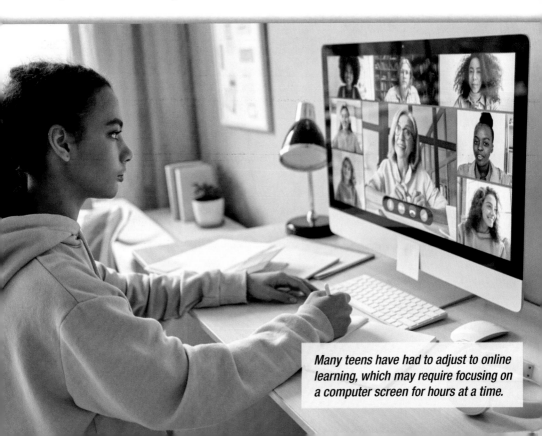

Many teens have had to adjust to online learning, which may require focusing on a computer screen for hours at a time.

doing a study-abroad program in Italy and had recently started a romance with a new partner. Then the coronavirus pandemic surged in Europe. Abruptly, the study abroad program shut down, and Suntheimer returned to the United States to quarantine, without her partner. At home, she sank into a depression. "I no longer had classes to keep me occupied. I'm missing my partner horribly in Italy, and there's no hope of getting back soon," Suntheimer says. Like many of her peers, Suntheimer has been dealing with the shift to virtual classes and a demanding workload. She has also been trying to prepare for a future that is uncertain and changing. "As a person who's going to graduate in two years, I see absolutely no certainty in what the world will look like in two years,"[47] Suntheimer says.

According to mental health experts, that uncertainty can be psychologically damaging to young people. "College students were particularly vulnerable because just about every college and university in the country sent everyone home. So imagine losing your job, your housing, your classes, your peer group—you lost everything overnight,"[48] says Kent State psychology researcher Joel Hughes. COVID-19 has increased stressors for already stressed-out teens and young adults, heightening the risk of anxiety, depression, and other mental health problems.

Extreme anxiety can disrupt sleep, and lack of sleep can increase anxiety. This cycle is familiar to Kayla Monnette. Monnette is a sophomore at the University of California, San Diego. The coronavirus pandemic has made her so anxious that she has trouble sleeping. "Whenever I go to sleep, I get a terrible feeling in my stomach and I can't sleep,"[49] she says. Monnette believes the stress of moving to online classes and worrying about high-

> "College students were particularly vulnerable because just about every college and university in the country sent everyone home. So imagine losing your job, your housing, your classes, your peer group—you lost everything overnight."[48]
>
> —Joel Hughes, a psychology researcher at Kent State University

Create a Friend "Pod"

For teens and young adults, the isolation and loneliness caused by the pandemic has been challenging to manage. To help young people overcome these feelings, some psychologists have recommended that teens and young adults create small "pods" of a few friends who agree to follow strict safety rules, both when they are together and apart. This allows people in the pod to socialize safely with each other and reduce the risk of getting or spreading the coronavirus. According to Anne Marie Albano, a medical psychology professor at Columbia University Irving Medical Center in New York, having a friend pod has given young people a way to meet their need for social interaction safely.

risk family members has contributed to her persistent anxiety. Not knowing how many people on campus were infected also added to Monnette's fears of getting sick herself. Eventually, she decided to move into an off-campus apartment, where she would be in contact with fewer people and have a lower risk of becoming infected. The move helped ease some of her stress. "I think a huge contribution to my anxiety was the insecure and temporary feeling that being on campus [during a pandemic] gave me,"[50] she says.

Searching for Support

At a time when mental health challenges have been rising, some of the usual resources for teens and young adults have been less available. In some cases parents, teachers, and other adult mentors have been preoccupied with their own troubles and have not been able to provide support and advice. Also, many traditional in-person mental health services have been shut down or moved online. While some people find online counseling helpful, others struggle without in-person support. When Valerie Johnson, a senior at the University of California, Berkeley, experienced some mental health issues, she decided to visit campus counseling. When she found out the appointment would be online, she decided not to schedule a visit. "I don't see myself doing well in an online [therapy] environment because I can barely show up to online classes," Johnson says. "I don't think I would benefit the same as in-person. I feed off other people's energy, eye contact, and body language."[51]

While the coronavirus has made it more difficult for teens and young adults to get help, the stigma surrounding mental health counseling and support has lessened. Because mental health in relation to the pandemic is now being discussed more frequently and new types of online resources are being offered, it is becoming more accepted for young people to admit they need help and seek it out. "The hopeful piece for me is it seems like we're at an inflection point. All of a sudden, it's OK to talk about mental health,"[52] says Kelly Davis, director of peer advocacy support and services for Mental Health America.

Turning to Unhealthy Behaviors

Without their usual support networks, some teens and young adults have turned to unhealthy behaviors to cope with stress, depression, and anxiety. According to the August 2020 CDC report on mental health during the pandemic, 25 percent of young adults reported they had started or increased substance use to cope with stress and difficult emotions. A separate study of adolescents, published in the September 2020 *Journal of Adolescent Health*, found that although the percentage of teens using substances declined during the pandemic, those who did use alcohol and marijuana said they used these substances more frequently. "The isolation has scared a lot of people—for anyone, the unknown is very scary, and teens and adolescents, the unknown has scared them," says Latrice Mason, a therapist who specializes in substance-use disorders among teenagers. "They're looking for an escape, something that helps them feel good, because socialization has been a big part of their lives, and that's not true anymore."[53]

Substance abuse is even more concerning because it can magnify suicidal feelings. Suicide risk can be linked to impulsiveness, explains Dr. Sarah Vinson, an associate professor of psychiatry and pediatrics at Morehouse School of Medicine.

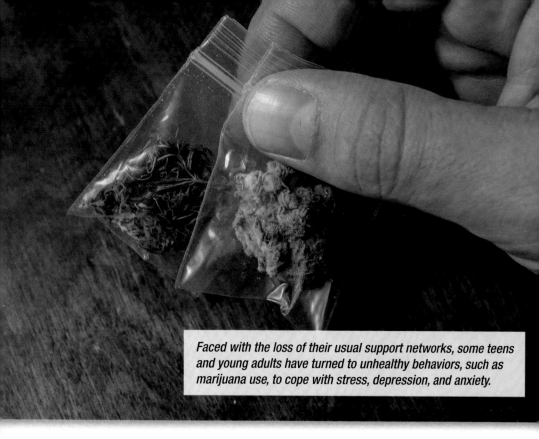

Faced with the loss of their usual support networks, some teens and young adults have turned to unhealthy behaviors, such as marijuana use, to cope with stress, depression, and anxiety.

"We know people will often act more impulsively if they are using substances, which exacerbate mental health issues,"[54] she says. While this is always a worry, it has stood out during the pandemic. According to the CDC, one in four young adults reported that they had seriously considered suicide since the start of the pandemic. The combination of uncertainty and worry about the future that has left many teens and young adults without much hope. "Hopelessness is one of the big drivers of suicide," says Vinson. "It's normally not about wanting to be dead; it's about not wanting to live like this, whatever *this* is."[55]

While people of all ages have been affected by the pandemic, teens and young adults have been hit particularly hard. People in this age group tends to rely heavily on social connections as they transition from adolescence to adulthood. Without engaging in their usual social activities, many teens and young adults have found themselves experiencing symptoms of anxiety, depression, and other mental health conditions.

CHAPTER FIVE

Dealing with Loss

Paula Bronstein traveled from Thailand, where she had been living, to the United States in March 2020 to say good-bye to her father, George Bronstein. George had lived a good, long life. At age 101, he was dying of natural causes. Paula prepared to say good-bye and be with him in his last days. However, the coronavirus pandemic changed her plans.

When Paula arrived in the United States, she self-quarantined and was not permitted to see her father in person. When George died on March 30, his daughter was not allowed to be with him. After his death, she and other family members and friends were not allowed to gather for the traditional Jewish rituals or for a funeral service. Instead, only a few family members were permitted to attend the burial, as long as they stayed in their cars. Only the rabbi was allowed to stand at the grave site and perform the Jewish custom of tossing a shovelful of dirt onto the casket. Paula sat nearby in a rented car so that she could hear the prayers and other words spoken by the rabbi. As a photojournalist who has documented wars, earthquakes, typhoons, and other disasters, Paula says of her job, "I've seen a lot—I've experienced horrific things." She says those experiences "didn't prepare me for sitting in a rental car by myself, having to watch my father's casket going to the grave. . . . We couldn't even stand in a circle around the grave at the proper social distance. It just caused so much pain for our family; it couldn't have been much worse." She believes that finding peace "is going to take a while because we just couldn't do it properly."[56]

Hundreds of thousands of people worldwide have died from COVID-19 and other ailments during the coronavirus pandemic. As Paula Bronstein's story illustrates, the coronavirus pandemic has disrupted sacred rituals and traditions around death and dying. This is changing how the people left behind grieve and process loss. Friends and loved ones who cannot grieve in the typical ways can be left with unresolved feelings of loss, pain, and guilt. Some may even feel responsible for their loved one's death. If these feelings are allowed to fester and grow, they can lead to mental health issues.

> "I've seen a lot—I've experienced horrific things. . . . [It] didn't prepare me for sitting in a rental car by myself, having to watch my father's casket going to the grave."[56]
>
> —Paula Bronstein, a photojournalist who was not able to give her father a traditional burial during the pandemic

A Solitary Death

Many people have a fear of dying alone. For too many people that fear has become reality. As deaths from COVID-19 spiraled out of control in the United States, hospitals, nursing homes, and senior-care facilities closed to visitors. In many cases family, friends, and clergy were not allowed to be with those who were sick and dying in their final hours. This absence can affect the dying as well as those left behind. Patients with COVID-19 were twelve times more likely to die in a medical facility where they could not have visitors as compared to patients who died of any cause in 2018, a July 2020 study found. Many of these patients were dying alone because of restrictions put in place to slow the spread of coronavirus during the pandemic. "Where you die is important and reflects end-of-life quality for the patient and the family," says lead author Dr. Sadiya Khan, a Northwestern Medicine physician. "The patients dying of COVID-19 in medical facilities may not have any family with them because of visitor restrictions."[57]

Not being able to be with a loved one at the end of life can be especially traumatic for surviving family members. Khan says:

A loved one dying alone takes a huge mental toll on families. It impairs the family's ability to grieve and cope with the loss. For patients, we've all thought about how terrible it would be to have to die alone. This is the horror happening to thousands of people in medical facilities where no family member or loved one is able to be present with them during their final moments on earth.[58]

In addition to not having family members at their bedside, those dying during the coronavirus pandemic have also not been allowed other end-of-life comforts and rituals. Hospital chaplains have been discouraged from spending time with dying patients or holding their hands to comfort them. Unable to enter medical facilities or patient rooms, Roman Catholic priests have not been able to administer the last rites to a dying person, which requires physical touch, giving the person communion, and anointing them with oil. Instead, some priests have tried to provide blessings to dying patients over the phone or from a hallway.

> "A loved one dying alone takes a huge mental toll on families. It impairs the family's ability to grieve and cope with the loss."[58]
>
> —Dr. Sadiya Khan, a Northwestern Medicine physician

Nurses and other health care workers have tried their best to comfort the dying and soothe the pain felt by family and friends. Fully gowned and masked, they have sat with dying patients until the patients have taken their last breaths. They have also helped family members see and speak to dying patients using webcams and cell phone video chat platforms. However, mental health experts say that it is simply not the same as being there in person.

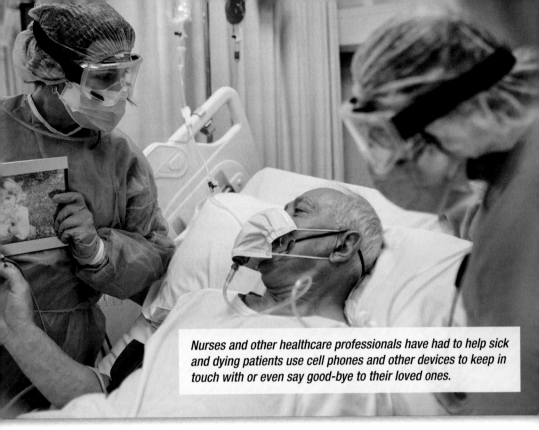

Nurses and other healthcare professionals have had to help sick and dying patients use cell phones and other devices to keep in touch with or even say good-bye to their loved ones.

Grieving Alone

Across a wide range of cultures and beliefs, when individuals die, their family, friends, and community process their death together. In most cultures funerals and memorial services allow friends and family to gather and to remember and celebrate the person who died, often by sharing fond memories. They allow survivors to remember the dead in a positive light and play an essential role in helping them navigate through the process of grief. "We cannot find anywhere a group of people in any era or any culture that has allowed the grieving to go it alone. The gathered community is essential to the grief process and the funeral process; it's as near a universal as we've got,"[59] says William Hoy, a clinical professor of medical humanities at Baylor University.

However, during the coronavirus pandemic, processing death has become a solitary event. Because many states and even countries have banned large gatherings and travel, few family and friends can physically attend funerals. For those who can

Ribbons of Remembrance Memorial

In Westchester County, New York, officials have created a new memorial called Ribbons of Remembrance, which is dedicated to county residents who have died from COVID-19. The memorial stands in a nature preserve overlooking the Hudson River. At the memorial, ribbons and permanent markers are available for visitors who wish to honor a loved one lost to COVID-19. Visitors can write the name of their loved one on the ribbon and tie it to one of two designated trees or a rope structure that is part of the memorial. "We need within our culture certain social points where we can come together," says County Executive George Latimer to explain why Westchester County decided to create the COVID-19 memorial. "We have all lost people that we know and love through this [pandemic]."

Quoted in ABC 7, "Coronavirus News: Westchester County Honors COVID-19 Victims with 'Ribbons of Remembrance,'" May 6, 2020. https://abc7ny.com.

be present, many traditional funeral rites and traditions cannot be performed. In New York, Muslim families have been forced to skip or alter the traditional bathing of the deceased, an essential Islamic death ritual. Islamic and Jewish traditions require the burial of the dead within twenty-four hours of death. Yet because morgues and funeral homes have been overwhelmed during the pandemic, some families have had to wait days to bury their loved ones. In Christian families traditional wakes to commemorate a person's life with family and friends have been canceled. Without these familiar rites and rituals, the surviving family may have difficulty processing their grief.

Complicated Grief

During the pandemic, many people have been able to adapt to the changes in death and mourning and experience the normal process of bereavement. They may still feel sadness or pain over the loss of their loved one but are able to return to daily life relatively quickly. They can work, go about their daily lives, and feel connected to others.

However, for others, the disruption to familiar grieving rituals during the pandemic has made it more difficult to process the loss of a loved one during the pandemic. For some people, being unable to mourn in the usual ways can trigger depression, anxiety, and other trauma disorders. In some cases a person may develop a mental health condition called prolonged grief disorder, also known as complicated grief. A person with complicated grief will be preoccupied with thoughts and memories of the deceased. Their emotional pain interferes with their ability to function and perform day-to-day activities. Complicated grief is different from normal feelings of grief and sadness and can last six months or more. "Complicated grief is an inability to accept the loss and move forward. The symptoms become debilitating and don't improve with time,"[60] says Dr. Divya Jose, a New York City psychiatrist.

In normal times, people have a greater risk of developing complicated grief if they have a history of mood and anxiety disorders or have experienced a prior trauma or loss. They may also be more likely to develop complicated grief if their loved

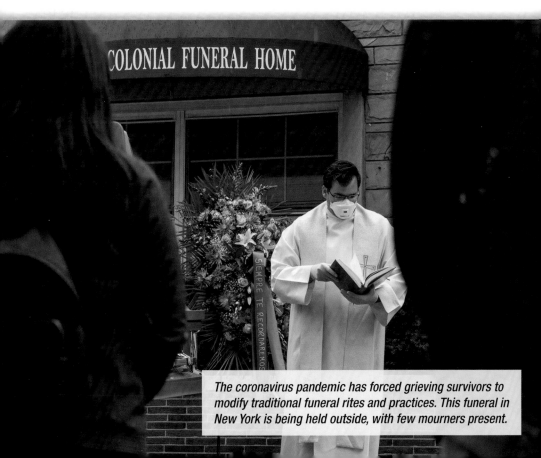

The coronavirus pandemic has forced grieving survivors to modify traditional funeral rites and practices. This funeral in New York is being held outside, with few mourners present.

Losing a loved one during the coronavirus pandemic can be extremely challenging. At certain times, grief can feel overwhelming. To cope with grief during the pandemic, mental health experts recommend various actions. First, it is important to try to make and maintain connections with other people. Invite others to share stories and pictures via letters, emails, phone calls, social media, or video calls. Host conference calls or Zoom chats with family and friends to stay connected. Another way to manage grief is to create memories or rituals about the loved one. Create a virtual memory book or web page about the person and ask family and friends to contribute to it. Do something that had special meaning to the loved one, such as preparing a favorite meal or making a favorite craft. It is also essential to reach out for help, such as grief counseling or mental health services if needed. Many services are offered over the phone or virtually when in-person meetings are not possible. Faith-based organizations and community groups can also provide support.

one experiences an unexpected or violent death, if they were the primary caregiver for their loved one before his or her death, or if they do not have social support after their loved one's death.

Because the pandemic has changed how many people experience death and disrupted its related rituals, mental health experts say that more people may be struggling with complicated grief. "In addition to the unexpected nature of coronavirus-related deaths, the disruption in traditional grieving processes—such as the practice of religious rituals, the limitation of visitors and the practice of social isolation—could potentially interfere with normal grieving, causing a rise in complicated grief,"[61] Jose says. Mental health experts caution that recognizing prolonged grief disorder is essential, because if left untreated, it can lead to more serious mental health problems, reduced quality of life, substance use, and even suicide.

> "The disruption in traditional grieving processes—such as the practice of religious rituals, the limitation of visitors and the practice of social isolation—could potentially interfere with normal grieving, causing a rise in complicated grief."[61]
>
> —Dr. Divya Jose, a psychiatrist in New York City

Filled with Guilt

In some cases feelings of loss have been amplified by feelings of guilt and worry. Some survivors have wondered why they survived the virus when another person died. Some have also worried that they unknowingly infected a loved one. Early in the pandemic, it was unknown how the virus passed from person to person. Even as scientists learned more about the virus, many uncertainties about transmission remained. The latest research shows that people who are infected with the coronavirus can be infectious and spread the virus for several days before they show symptoms or even know they have been infected. Even more troubling, many people are asymptomatic carriers of the virus, meaning they never develop symptoms but can spread the virus to others.

Sometimes survivors hold themselves responsible for family and friends who get sick. They beat themselves up over decisions they made that may have led to others getting infected with the virus and dying. At first, fifty-five-year-old Paul Stewart thought he simply had a bad cold. He did not think he could have the coronavirus, even

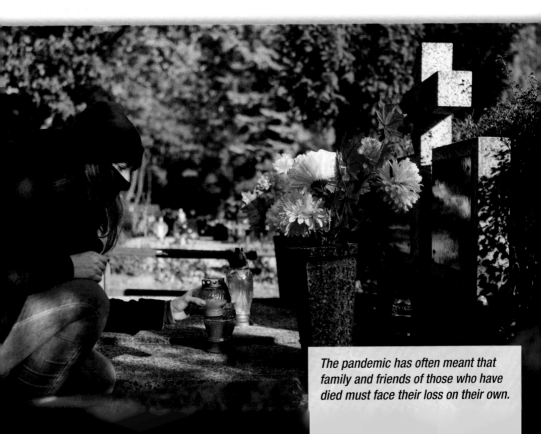

The pandemic has often meant that family and friends of those who have died must face their loss on their own.

after a coworker at the clinic where he worked as a rehabilitation technician tested positive. Then Paul's father, eighty-six-year-old Robert Stewart, appeared to have caught the same cold. For Robert, however, the cold got worse. Eventually, he became so ill that he passed out in the bathroom, and Paul called for an ambulance. At the hospital, Robert tested positive for the coronavirus. Paul suddenly wondered whether his cold was something more and he was to blame for his father's illness. "Could I have been more careful with what I thought was the common cold?" he asks. "If you felt the way I did now, you would not expose people to that. But there just wasn't enough information then. That's what I've struggled with."[62]

In the hospital, Robert began to fail, and doctors could do little to help him. Visitors were not permitted, and Paul never saw his father again in person before he died. Upon learning of his father's death, Paul told his girlfriend, "I just killed my dad. I gave this to my dad." Although others reassured him that his father's death was not his fault, Paul still struggled with guilt. "It's an odd feeling, like you're not at peace," he says. "You can't get rest because you're still dealing with the guilt." He kept wondering if he could have done something different. Would his father still be alive if he had quarantined in his bedroom, sanitized their home better, or taken his father to the hospital earlier? "I think about it every day," he says. "Could I have been more careful?"[63]

> "It's an odd feeling, like you're not at peace. You can't get rest because you're still dealing with the guilt."[63]
>
> —Paul Stewart, a man who struggles with guilt over whether he infected his father with COVID-19

The coronavirus pandemic has changed the way people worldwide deal with dying, death, and mourning. For many, the familiar rites and rituals of death cannot be performed, leaving the survivors to deal with their loss on their own. While losing a person we love and care about is always difficult, the pandemic has made it more challenging for the living to process their feelings. These lingering feelings can affect mental health and lead to anxiety, depression, and other mental health conditions.

Introduction: Missing Life

1. Quoted in Colleen Grablick, "Washingtonians Who Live Alone Are Feeling Depressed and Scared During the Pandemic," DCist, August 14, 2020. https://dcist.com.
2. Quoted in Grablick, "Washingtonians Who Live Alone Are Feeling Depressed and Scared During the Pandemic."
3. Quoted in Mental Health America, "Number of People Reporting Anxiety and Depression Nationwide Since the Start of Pandemic Hits All-Time High in September, Hitting Young People Hardest," October 20, 2020. www.mhanational.org.
4. Quoted in UN News, "COVID-19 Disrupting Critical Mental Health Services, WHO Warns," October 5, 2020. https://news.un.org.

Chapter One: Isolated and Lonely

5. Quoted in Chelsea Cirruzzo, "Pandemic Depression Is About to Collide with Seasonal Depression. Make a Plan, Experts Say," *Washington Post*, October 27, 2020. www.washingtonpost.com.
6. Quoted in Cirruzzo, "Pandemic Depression Is About to Collide with Seasonal Depression."
7. Quoted in Sharp, "Managing Loneliness During Covid-19," September 8, 2020. www.sharp.com.
8. Quoted in Ammar Kalia, "The Extreme Loneliness of Lockdown: 'Even Though My Partner Is Here, I'm Struggling to Cope,'" *The Guardian* (Manchester, UK), April 28, 2020. www.theguardian.com.
9. Quoted in Ashley Laderer, "What It's Like to Experience Depression for the First Time, in a Pandemic," Elemental, October 29, 2020. https://elemental.medium.com.
10. Quoted in Lynn Jolicoeur and Lisa Mullins, "Depression Increases More than Three-Fold in Wake of Pandemic, BU Study Finds," WBUR, September 2, 2020. www.wbur.org.
11. Quoted in Lindsey Tanner, "Depression, Anxiety Spike amid Outbreak and Turbulent Times," Associated Press, September 2, 2020. https://apnews.com.
12. Quoted in Tanner, "Depression, Anxiety Spike amid Outbreak and Turbulent Times."

13. Quoted in Laderer, "What It's Like to Experience Depression for the First Time, in a Pandemic."

14. Quoted in Arlene Borenstein, "Coronavirus Pandemic Causing Anxiety, Panic Attacks for Many," NBC Miami, May 14, 2020. www.nbc miami.com.

15. Quoted in Borenstein, "Coronavirus Pandemic Causing Anxiety, Panic Attacks for Many."

16. Quoted in Paige Minemyer, "GoodRX: COVID-19 Worsening Behavioral Health Concerns," Fierce Healthcare, December 14, 2020. www.fiercehealthcare.com.

17. Quoted in Scripps, "How to Stay Socially Connected While Social Distancing," April 17, 2020. www.scripps.org.

18. Allie Ouendag, "Zoom Friendships: Staying Connected in a Time of Social Distancing," *The Collegiate* (Grand Rapids, MI, Community College student newspaper), May 17, 2020. https://thecollegiate live.com.

19. Quoted in Pamela O'Brien, "How to Beat Loneliness in the Time of Social Distancing," *Shape*, October 22, 2020. www.shape.com.

Chapter Two: Money Worries

20. Chan Tran, "I Lost My Job Because of Coronavirus—Now What?," Northwell Health, 2020. https://thewell.northwell.edu.

21. Tran, "I Lost My Job Because of Coronavirus—Now What?"

22. Quoted in Ryan Coulter, "2 More Mountain Businesses Forced to Close Because of Pandemic," WLOS.com, October 28, 2020. https://wlos.com.

23. Quoted in Rhitu Chatterjee, "Juggling Financial Stress and Caregiving, Parents Are 'Very Not OK' in the Pandemic," New Orleans Public Radio, September 30, 2020. www.wwno.org.

24. Quoted in Chatterjee, "Juggling Financial Stress and Caregiving, Parents Are 'Very Not OK' in the Pandemic."

25. Quoted in Beth Adams, "Rochester's Unemployed: A Single Mother Tries to Adjust After Losing Her Job in the Pandemic," WXXI News, June 23, 2020. www.wxxinews.org.

26. Quoted in Adams, "Rochester's Unemployed."

27. Quoted in Stephanie Pappas, "The Toll of Job Loss," American Psychological Association, October 1, 2020. www.apa.org.

28. Quoted in Kristen Dalli, "Anxiety About Job Security and Finances Have Increased During the Pandemic," Consumer Affairs, September 25, 2020. www.consumeraffairs.com.

29. Quoted in Sasha Pezenik, "Alcohol Consumption Rising Sharply During Pandemic, Especially Among Women," ABC News, September 29, 2020. https://abcnews.go.com.

30. Quoted in Pezenik, "Alcohol Consumption Rising Sharply During Pandemic, Especially Among Women."
31. Quoted in Pezenik, "Alcohol Consumption Rising Sharply During Pandemic, Especially Among Women."

Chapter Three: The Mental Health Toll on Essential Workers

32. Quoted in Meghan McCarty Carino, "Essential Workers Pressured by Mental Health Issues," Marketplace, August 14, 2020. www.marketplace.org.
33. Jess, "Coping with Anxiety After Getting Covid-19: A Nurse's Story," Mind, May 19, 2020. www.mind.org.uk.
34. Quoted in Michael Sainato, "'I Cry Before Work': US Essential Workers Burned Out amid Pandemic," The Guardian (Manchester, UK), September 23, 2020. www.theguardian.com.
35. Quoted in Sainato, "'I Cry Before Work.'"
36. Quoted in Bryn Nelson and David B. Kaminsky, "Covid-19's Crushing Mental Health Toll on Health Care Workers," American Cancer Society Journals, September 4, 2020. https://acsjournals.online library.wiley.com.
37. Quoted in Giulia McDonnell Nieto del Rio, "'I Can Never Do Enough': I.C.U. Workers Record Their Anguish as the Coronavirus Surges," New York Times, October 28, 2020. www.nytimes.com.
38. Quoted in del Rio, "'I Can Never Do Enough.'"
39. Quoted in Jan Hoffman, "'I Can't Turn My Brain Off': PTSD and Burnout Threaten Medical Workers," New York Times, May 16, 2020. www.nytimes.com.
40. Quoted in Hoffman, "'I Can't Turn My Brain Off.'"
41. Quoted in Hoffman, "'I Can't Turn My Brain Off.'"

Chapter Four: Vulnerable Teens and Young Adults

42. Quoted in Emma Goldberg, "Teens in Covid Isolation: 'I Felt like I Was Suffocating,'" New York Times, November 12, 2020. www.nytimes.com.
43. Quoted in Goldberg, "Teens in Covid Isolation."
44. Quoted in Mayline Ruiz, "San Jose Students' Anxiety on the Rise with Pandemic," San Jose (CA) Mercury News, July 3, 2020. www.mercurynews.com.
45. Quoted in Goldberg, "Teens in Covid Isolation."
46. Quoted in Greta Anderson, "Students Reporting Depression and Anxiety at Higher Rates," Inside Higher Ed, August 19, 2020. www.insidehighered.com.

47. Quoted in Jeff St. Clair, "The Psychological Effects of the Pandemic Have Hit Young People Especially Hard," WKSU, October 15, 2020. www.wksu.org.
48. Quoted in St. Clair, "The Psychological Effects of the Pandemic Have Hit Young People Especially Hard."
49. Quoted in Ethan Edward Coston, "Pandemic Tests an Already Fragile College Mental Health System," CalMatters, August 27, 2020. https://calmatters.org.
50. Quoted in Coston, "Pandemic Tests an Already Fragile College Mental Health System."
51. Quoted in Coston, "Pandemic Tests an Already Fragile College Mental Health System."
52. Quoted in Anderson, "Students Reporting Depression and Anxiety at Higher Rates."
53. Quoted in Aubrey Whelan and Bethany Ao, "Pandemic Isolation Has Some Teens Turning to Substance Use. Philly's Recovery High School Has Found Ways to Fight Back," *Philadelphia Inquirer*, September 8, 2020. www.inquirer.com.
54. Quoted in Perri Klass, "Young Adults' Pandemic Mental Health Risks," *New York Times*, August 24, 2020. www.nytimes.com.
55. Quoted in Klass, "Young Adults' Pandemic Mental Health Risks."

Chapter Five: Dealing with Loss

56. Quoted in Craig Welch, "How Should We Mourn When Coronavirus Keeps Us Apart?," National Geographic, April 16, 2020. www.nationalgeographic.com.
57. Quoted in Marla Paul, "More Lonely Deaths in Hospitals and Nursing Homes from COVID," Northwestern University, July 17, 2020. https://news.northwestern.edu.
58. Quoted in Paul, "More Lonely Deaths in Hospitals and Nursing Homes from COVID."
59. Quoted in Claire Felter et al., "How the World Has Learned to Grieve in a Pandemic," Council on Foreign Relations, May 19, 2020. www.cfr.org.
60. Quoted in Yalda Safai, "Covid-19 Deaths May Lead to Prolonged Grief Disorder," ABC News, July 9, 2020. https://abcnews.go.com.
61. Quoted in Safai, "Covid-19 Deaths May Lead to Prolonged Grief Disorder."
62. Quoted in Jon Schuppe, "'I Gave This to My Dad': COVID-19 Survivors Grapple with Guilt of Infecting Family," NBC News, May 16, 2020. www.nbcnews.com.
63. Quoted in Schuppe, "'I Gave This to My Dad.'"

American Psychiatric Association

www.psychiatry.org

The American Psychiatric Association is an organization of member physicians working together to ensure human care and effective treatment for all persons with mental disorders. Its website includes a COVID-19 information hub with a special section on mental health resources for families.

American Psychological Association

www.apa.org

The American Psychological Association represents American psychologists, who study and treat human behavior. The association's website features a special page of COVID-19 resources for psychologists, health care workers, and the general public at www.apa.org/topics/covid-19.

Centers for Disease Control and Prevention (CDC)

www.cdc.gov

The CDC is the premier public health agency in the United States. Its website includes the latest information about the coronavirus and COVID-19. The website also has a useful section about coping with stress during the pandemic. Links to articles and where to get help can be found at www.cdc.gov/coronavirus/2019-ncov/daily-life-coping/managing-stress-anxiety.html.

Mental Health America

www.mhanational.org

Mental Health America is an advocacy group for people with mental illnesses and their families. Its website features many resources, including an interactive tool to assist in finding mental health help, information on support groups, and mental health screening tools.

National Alliance on Mental Illness (NAMI)

www.nami.org

NAMI is an advocacy group for people with mental illnesses and has local chapters across the country. Its website offers a variety of resources, including information about mental health conditions, support groups, help lines, and more. There is also a special section focused on information for frontline professionals at www.nami.org/Your-Journey/Frontline-Professionals.

National Institute of Mental Health (NIMH)
www.nimh.nih.gov

The NIMH is the federal government's chief funding agency for mental health research in America. The institute's website provides a variety of information, including a special section of resources to help in coping with COVID-19 at www.nimh.nih.gov/health/education-awareness/shareable-resources-on-coping-with-covid-19.shtml.

National Suicide Prevention Lifeline
https://suicidepreventionlifeline.org

The National Suicide Prevention Lifeline provides free, confidential support for people in distress. The toll-free number is 800-273-8255. Help is available 24/7. The website includes information and resources for people who are struggling with the COVID-19 pandemic. It also has sections aimed at youth, Native Americans, LGBTQ individuals, and other groups.

US Department of Health and Human Services (HHS)
www.hhs.gov

The HHS is a department of the federal government that strives to protect the health of all Americans and provide essential human services. Its website has the latest information about the coronavirus and COVID-19. It also has a section dealing with mental health and coping with the pandemic at www.hhs.gov/coronavirus/mental-health-and-coping/index.html.

World Health Organization (WHO)
www.who.int

The WHO is an agency of the United Nations that is responsible for international public health. Its website has the latest information about the coronavirus and COVID-19.

Books

Andrea Balinson, *Depression, Anxiety, and Bipolar Disorders*. Broomall, PA: Mason Crest, 2017.

A.W. Buckey, *Dealing with Anxiety Disorder*. San Diego: Reference-Point, 2020.

Tabatha Chansard, *Conquer Anxiety Workbook for Teens: Find Peace from Worry, Panic, Fear, and Phobias*. Emeryville, CA: Althea, 2019.

Hal Marcovitz. *The COVID-19 Pandemic: The World Turned Upside Down*. San Diego: ReferencePoint, 2020.

Albert Marrin, *Very, Very, Very Dreadful: The Influenza Pandemic of 1918*. New York: Knopf Books for Young Readers, 2018.

Internet Sources

Mathiew Desnard et al., "COVID-19 Job and Income Loss Leading to More Hunger and Financial Hardship," Brookings Institution, July 13, 2020. www.brookings.edu.

Kira M. Newman, "Seven Ways the Pandemic Is Affecting Our Mental Health," *Greater Good Magazine*, August 11, 2020. www.greatergood.berkeley.edu.

Kim Parker et al., "Economic Fallout from COVID-19 Continues to Hit Lower-Income Americans the Hardest," Pew Research Center, September 24, 2020. www.pewsocialtrends.org.

Maddy Savage, "Coronavirus: The Possible Long-Term Mental Health Impacts," BBC, October 28, 2020. www.bbc.com.

INDEX